Nutrition

How to Eat for Wellness and Fitness

By
Bring On Fitness

About Bring On Fitness

Our passion for fitness gave life to **Bring On Fitness**. We started with the goal of helping as many people as we can. To educate, motivate and to help change peoples lives for the better. Bring On Fitness is not only for the fitness enthusiasts, but also for the beginner. We strongly believe nothing is more important than learning the basics and creating a strong foundation in both nutrition - through meal planning, and in exercise - by following a specific plan. This is just as important for the beginner, as it is for the experienced athlete.

We set high standards for ourselves, the information we share, and the products we carry. Our goal is to provide you with exceptional products that suit your needs and the knowledge and motivation to help you work towards and achieve your health and fitness goals.

Check us out at www.bringonfitness.com

"Our Mission is to have a positive impact in changing peoples lives. We will deliver the best possible fitness and nutrition solutions that will empower people to achieve their health and fitness goals."

Table of Contents

About Bring On Fitness 5

Introduction 9

Chapter 1: Understanding the Basics .... .11

Calorie Equation..11

Source of Calories...12

Carbohydrates..12

Fats 13

Proteins...14

Vitamins..15

Minerals..15

Water 16

Probiotics...17

Chapter 2: Role of a Balanced Diet in Weight Loss and Nutrition... .19

Colorful Meals...20

Water as a Savior..20

Moderation is the Key..21

Sugar, Salt, and Everything Nice.............................21

Chapter 3: How to Get the Most Nutrients Out of your Food...23

Pairing Smart..23

A little Fat with that Vitamins Please 23

Pairing Iron with Vitamin C...24

Pairing Zinc and Iron with Sulfur 24

Straight from the Earth...24

Chop, Blend, Crush, Soak..25

Retaining the Nutrients...25

Storing...25

Eating raw 26

Cooking 26

Chapter 4: Exercise or Diet: What matters more? .. 27

Conclusion
.... .2
9

Introduction

I want to thank you for choosing this book, "*Nutrition: How to Eat for Wellness and Fitness.*"

With the improvements in our standard of living over the years, we have more choices in every aspect of our lives. Whether in food, fashion, lifestyle, and living, we are presented with more and more options everywhere. When it comes to food, which forms a fundamental part of our lives, we have quite a variety to choose from. However, using this freedom that we have in the right way is becoming more of an issue. Taste is overpowering our sense of judgement.

Temporary satisfaction of the palate is the only thing that is of concern now; health and nutrition are secondary. We hear of new diseases every day – things that were unheard of back in the good old days. People are struggling for a good physique by resorting to wrong eating habits, from anorexia to bulimia.

Obesity levels across the world are on the rise, and this has led to more and more cases of depression and bullying, especially among the teens; body shaming and suicides are what results out of all this.

The pressure on body organs is also increasing with increasing weight. Cardiovascular disease is a common health issue now. The medical funds of the government are being used to treat disorders, which arise out of the lifestyles of the people and which could easily be prevented by a balanced diet and self-control.

Measures like short-duration heavy gym activity and crash diets are what people turn to. We need to realize that these short-term measures – while they give results quickly – are exactly what they are, i.e., short lived. It takes an ugly turn when these measures backfire badly. Instead, a balanced and healthy diet should be adopted, along with light exercises that are easy to stick to so that the body is not put under unnecessary strain and remains fit.

All people have their own perspective of what wellness is. It has never been easier to harm ourselves with the food that we eat and, at the same time, it has never been easier to heal ourselves. Most people know that a good diet, sleep, and exercise are the cornerstones of health but are confused about how to go about it.

Low-fat, low-carb, plant-based, Paleo, raw-food, vegetarian, or vegan diets present too many choices. There is no one right way and thus, to each his or her own. In short, all of us are unique. You just have to find the balance and make sure it's on your own terms, with your specific goals and values in mind. An objective, a plan, and tactics are all you need, and you are set to start your wellness journey.

So what is nutrition? It is, in fact, the process of providing the body with food that is required for proper growth and health. Whether you are a teenager, an athlete, or a person who is overweight and wants to lead a better and healthier life, nutrition is what will get you there. Great nutrition boosts the performance of athletes, helps in the healthy growth of teenagers, and also helps overweight people eat healthier and achieve their weight goals.

Thanks again for purchasing this book. I hope you enjoy it!

Chapter 1: Understanding the Basics

Calorie Equation

The Calorie Equation is a simple concept. When the outflow is more than the inflow, we get a deficit; similarly, when the calorie expenditure is more than the calorie intake, a calorie deficit is created, which leads to successful weight loss. Everything that we consume by way of eating or drinking (except for water) has a calorific value. Calories are what are used by our body as a source of energy to complete its daily functions.

Consuming more calories than what is used leads to surplus calories, which, in turn, get stored as fat in the body. When there is a calorie deficit, it is this fat that the body breaks down to release energy, as the calories that were supplied have already been used; this leads to the slimming of the body.

Our body is fueled by calories, so it does not mean that calorie intake should be stopped completely in order to lose weight. Even when we are not doing any heavy physical activities, calories are needed to maintain all the vital functions of our body, such as brain functioning, pumping of blood, building cartilage, bone and nervous system tissues and breathing.

When there is a scarcity of calories, the body becomes weak and thus becomes prone to health risks and disease. Moreover, starvation leads to weight gain rather than weight loss. This is because when the amount of calories is drastically limited, our body switches to starvation mode. Whatever calories come in get stored in the form of fat in body tissues. In this scenario, even if a small diet is taken after a prolonged period of starvation, it gets converted into fat, which leads to obesity.

Source of Calories

The source from which calories are obtained is equally important. Glucose is the ultimate source of energy in our body. Every nutritional component that we eat or drink is ultimately converted into glucose.

The sources can mainly be divided into two areas: macronutrients and micronutrients. Macronutrients are basically what our body requires in large quantities to grow, repair, develop, and feel good. These include carbohydrates, fats, and proteins. Micronutrients are equally important. However, as their name suggests, they are required only in smaller quantities. They include mainly vitamins and minerals.

Some of the main nutritional components that affect weight loss or gain are mentioned below.

Carbohydrates

Carbohydrates come from legumes, grains, bread, dairy products, pasta, fruits, and vegetables. Depending on their molecular structure, they are either classified as simple or complex. Carbohydrates comprise 45% to 65% of the total daily calorie intake and provide 4 calories per gram. When digested, carbohydrates are broken down into simple sugars, commonly called glucose, which is then used by the body in multiple ways. Whatever extra is there is then converted into glycogen and stored for later use in the liver.

However, not all carbohydrates are equal; there are good and bad sources. Good carbohydrate sources are those that have complex carbohydrates. These aid in the slow release of glucose and remain in the body for quite a long time. Some good choices include brown rice, lentils, barley, oatmeal cookies, raisin bran, angel food cake, sweet potatoes, and couscous.

By eating whole grains and products made from these unrefined grains, you can enjoy the benefit of nutrients and fiber that are usually removed during the refining process. Bad carbohydrates are those which increase the glucose level in the blood for a short duration of time. Such sudden increases in the blood glucose level is harmful to the body as it, in turn, leads to insulin spikes, and as this glucose does not last long, the body then runs out of energy quicker. This leads to fatigue and hunger, which leaves you craving for more carbohydrates, consequently creating a vicious cycle.

However, carbohydrates are not to be avoided completely. They are the only source of fuel for many organs, like the kidneys and brain. In its absence, the body starts to rely on other sources of energy like proteins, which leads to the over production of ketone bodies that lead to the disruption of the body's metabolism.

Fats

A lot of people assume that fats are bad. All fats do not necessarily have a negative impact on our body. Fats are an important part of our diets as well. Fats are used by our body to form the major part of all cell membranes. Moreover, fats play an essential role in the absorption of certain vitamins. According to the USDA dietary guideline, 25% to 30% of our calories should come from fats, which provide about 9 calories per gram. Similar to carbohydrates, the important point here is to differentiate between the good and bad sources of fats and to stay away from the bad ones.

The best choices are unsaturated fats: Mono Unsaturated Fatty Acids (MUFA) and Poly Unsaturated Fatty Acids (PUFA). They help prevent the formation of plaque in the arteries and raise good cholesterol levels in our body. Monounsaturated fats are found in plant oils, pecans, avocados, and peanuts, whereas polyunsaturated fats are found in tuna, salmon, lobster, and corn and sunflower oils. Processed trans fats and saturated fats should be avoided. These are the major culprits behind the spread of obesity and also the cause of inflammation in the body; they also promote heart disease. Trans fats are primarily present in junk food like chips, fries, crackers, and cakes.

However, under-consumption of fats actually slows weight loss. This tends to affect the metabolism-boosting hormone that's released from the fat cells, which leads to the slowing down of metabolism and, in turn, leading to weight gain.

Proteins

About 15% to 20% percent of our calories should come from protein sources each day, like carbohydrates. They also contain about 4 calories per gram, say the USDA dietary guidelines. Most of the protein gets converted to glucose. It takes around three to five hours to release glucose, which makes it a smart source of calories.

Most proteins get stored in the muscle cells, which aids in bodybuilding. All this makes it a favored source of calories, and people try to replace other sources of energy with proteins. However, overconsumption of proteins also has side effects. Most of the high-protein food sources like dairy and meat are also high in saturated fat that leads to weight gain. Ketone bodies are produced on protein metabolism, and too much of them damages the body.

In America, meat is a primary source of protein, but plant sources are also available, such as legumes, seeds, nuts, and grains. Plant sources, with the exception of soy, must be combined with other foods, as they do not provide all of the amino acids that our bodies require to function normally.

Vitamins

Vitamins help our bodies by boosting the immune system and healing wounds. They also assist the body in creating energy and repairing cellular damage. Vitamin C is essential to help with synthesizing collagen. Collagen is what helps the blood vessels form their structure and also your ligaments and bones. Common sources of vitamin C are citrus fruits, peppers, and strawberries. Folate is also essential in helping prevent birth defects, and women planning to become pregnant or who are pregnant should ideally be taking folic acid supplements, which is the man-made form of folate, after consulting their doctor. Similarly, Vitamin D is essential to maintain calcium homeostasis, and this is naturally absorbed from the sun or certain foods.

Minerals

Minerals are important for proper body function and nutrition. They are important for nerve functions, muscles, hair and skin, and also for bone formation. Minerals also help with metabolic functions that help to convert food into energy. One of the main minerals that our body needs is sodium; as it helps to maintain the volume of fluid outside the cell and also helps the muscles to function normally. Excess of sodium, in salt form, is dangerous, and it can cause fluid retention, which leads to weight gain. Potassium is another mineral that helps maintain fluid levels outside and inside the cells and also prevents a rise in blood pressure associated with increased sodium intake. The best sources of potassium are tomatoes, potatoes, and bananas. Calcium is also needed to maintain and promote the growth of bones and teeth, and it is best to take at least three servings a day in the form of yoghurt, cheese, and milk.

Water

Water is one of the most important substances in the world and a universal solvent for the human body; it helps to transport essential nutrients to our cells. It hydrates the body and also acts as a lubricant during the process of digestion. A human body can survive longer without food than it can without water. Dehydration is one of the biggest causes of problems in the body, as it leads to a disruption in the efficient transportation of nutrients. All foods and drinks that are high in moisture content can be counted toward your intake of water. This includes soup, cucumber, and watermelon. These should be made a regular part of your diet. An adult is required to take about two to three liters of water every day or between 20 and 35 milliliters of water per kilogram of their body weight.

Probiotics

This is a word that is often associated with dietary supplements that have adequate amounts of gut friendly bacteria in them. These beneficial microorganisms, provided they are in the right amounts, help the digestive system work properly. An imbalance is created in the intestinal flora when we consume a diet rich in processed foods and sugar but low in vegetables and fresh fruit. It is even more disturbed when antibiotics are added to this already imbalanced mixture. Moreover, chicken, beef, eggs, and cow's milk all work toward killing off beneficial bacteria. This upsets the digestive system and causes irregular bowel movements. Probiotics can also be sourced from kefir, yoghurt, and other forms of cultured dairy products.

Chapter 2: Role of a Balanced Diet in Weight Loss and Nutrition

It can be tempting to replace one source of nutrient completely with another. However, depending on only one source hinders the journey to health. All the nutritional components are required to be in a balance to achieve this. Over consumption of just one nutrient can hinder weight loss and harms the body.

A lot of different kinds of fad diets are commonly practiced today that suggest cutting down on one type of nutrient source with the intention of fat loss. However, these kinds of diets are harmful in the long run. If we take an example, the same quantity of fat contains more calories than carbohydrate; there are lots of diets that cut down on fat and replace it with carbohydrates instead. This is, in fact, harmful to the body as it results in an insulin spike in the blood, which in turn makes it difficult for our body to access the fat stored for energy. Similarly, low-carbohydrate diets are not good.

In these cases, the body actually begins to release energy by using up stored glycogen. Water is required to release this glycogen energy in the ratio 3:1. Thus, the weight loss that is observed initially in these diets is primarily because of water loss.

A balance must be achieved between the major nutrient components to achieve weight loss. The question remains as to how to go about achieving this balance. There are also a lot of other micro and macronutrients that help in achieving health goals when taken in the right amounts. Items that will help you embark on this journey of a balanced diet are listed below.

Colorful Meals

Adding as many colors as possible to your plate will help you achieve your goals. Fruits and vegetables of every sort should be a part of your diet. The more colorful your meal, the better nutrition it will provide. It's hard to go wrong with fruit and vegetables as they contain only the required amounts of fats. Moreover, they contain fiber and complex carbohydrates, which all, in turn, contribute to weight loss. They also have natural sugars instead of processed sugars that are found in junk food, which also adds to their benefits. Apart from their role in helping with weight loss, they also have vitamins and antioxidants that help to improve metabolism and help boost our immune system. This, in turn, improves digestion and promotes weight loss. Make sure to choose whole fruit over juice, or else, you lose out on all the fiber, which helps with nutrient absorption.

Water as a Savior

When you feel hungry next time, just grab a glass of water. Most of the time, it's thirst that's mistaken for hunger. Our body finds it difficult to differentiate between hunger and thirst, and we end up overeating as a result. Moreover, drinking water about 30 minutes before a meal makes you feel fuller and helps you address the problem of overeating. Just make sure not to drink water while eating your meals or right after, as this leads to diluting gastric juices in the stomach, which slows down the digestion process. Slow digestion then leads to the slowing of your metabolism and putting on weight as a result.

Moderation is the Key

Include everything in your diet. Whites like wheat, rice, and cereals are all good to have but in limited quantities. They are an important source of fiber and carbohydrates for the body. However, over consumption can lead to weight gain. Moreover, it is best to avoid processed white flour at all costs. This provides calories but is devoid of fiber. Use wheat flour to make bread instead. Incorporating multigrain bread into your diet also gives your body a bunch of nutrients.

Sugar, Salt, and Everything Nice

Sugar has been recognized as a health threat. The addictive capacity of sugar has been proven by French scientists when the test rats chose sugar over cocaine, even while being addicted to cocaine. Sugar is difficult to stay away from, especially with ready meals and junk food that are readily available, as it is one of the key ingredients that add to the taste and oomph of everything that we eat.

Taste plays a major role in selling foods that have their fat levels lowered to convince people that they are, indeed, eating healthy. It was found that the sugar that was added was more potent and a leading cause of diabetes, obesity, and heart disease than any other sources of calories. The average can of soda packs about 10 to 12 teaspoons of sugar, and, considering that some people reach for more than a can or two in a day, it is no wonder that obesity has reached the current levels. It is to be noted that the total number of calories that we consume is actually irrelevant; it's the source of these calories that makes all the difference in the world.

We may think of how sodium might negatively affect our systems. As mentioned earlier, moderation is the key to nutrition. However, most of the sodium intake in our country comes from restaurant and processed foods. Most of the time, we do not know we are eating it, and too much of it, too. Salt helps to modify flavor and preserve foods; not all foods that contain salt appear to be salty, and there are so many variations of sodium that help to enhance flavors in different ways. Some affect water activity, but a lot of others affect the chemical reactions in food, preventing them from spoiling. Salt raises blood pressure, and this is what leads to heart failure, heart attacks, and strokes. There is also a lot of evidence to show that high salt intake and chances of stomach cancer, kidney disease, kidney stones, osteoporosis, water retention, and vascular dementia are correlated. Salt is essential in moderate amounts, but going overboard will eventually kill us.

Chapter 3: How to Get the Most Nutrients Out of your Food

There is a whole process behind eating – preparation, biting into the food, chewing it, and then digestion. There are a lot of chemical and mechanical changes that are brought about by these steps on the food that we eat. It affects the nutritional content of food and also the degree to which each of these nutrients will then be available for your body to absorb. Eating raw helps bring out and absorb the best when it comes to some nutrients, while for others, cooking, breaking down by crushing or cutting, or even eating them along with other foods brings out the best nutrients.

Pairing Smart

A little Fat with that Vitamins Please

Pairing Vitamins like A, D, E, and K with natural fats helps dissolve them and prepare them for easy absorption. However, you need to keep track of how much of these vitamins you consume as they get stored as fat in your liver, unlike water-soluble vitamins like C, B_{12}, Folic acid, and biotin that get flushed out of your system when there is too much of them. Pairing foods like carrots, squash, and sweet potatoes (Vitamin A), mushrooms and eggs (Vitamin D), Swiss chard, asparagus, and spinach (vitamin E), and spinach, broccoli, and kale (Vitamin K) with olive oil, coconut oil, avocado, mixed nuts, and/or butter gives you bonus points, and you will be scoring highly in this game of nutrition and healthy eating.

Pairing Iron with Vitamin C

Iron that we get from animal sources like dark poultry and red meat is called Heme Iron, whereas that we get from non-animal sources is called Nonheme Iron. Heme Iron is more readily available for absorption than Nonheme Iron; however, pairing them with Vitamin C helps increase their absorption.

Pairing foods like soybeans, spinach, kale, and lentils with some lemon juice, strawberries, orange slices, or chili peppers help you score some nutrients.

Pairing Zinc and Iron with Sulfur

It is best to eat foods rich in zinc and iron with sulfur-rich foods, as sulfur binds to these minerals and helps in their easy absorption. Therefore, foods like turkey, beef, and oysters (rich in zinc and iron) are best when paired with egg yolks, onion, and garlic.

Straight from the Earth

Plucking the fruit and vegetables from the soil separates them from the source of nutrients, and the longer they are away, the more nutrition they lose. Therefore, even the fresh fruit and vegetables that you buy from the stores will already have lost 20% to 60% of their nutrients unless you get them within four to five days of harvest. Growing your own fruit and vegetables also ensures that you get the most out of them.

Chop, Blend, Crush, Soak

These different kinds of food prep methods enhance the bioavailability of nutrients.

Chopping and crushing garlic and onion releases an enzyme called alliinase that helps form allicin. Allicin helps in the formation compounds that protect us against disease.

Soaking beans and grains reduces phytic acid, which otherwise blocks your absorption of calcium, zinc, and magnesium.

Cutting up vegetables and fruit helps in breaking down the plant cell walls and freeing up the nutrients.

Retaining the Nutrients

Storing

Oxygen, light, and heat degrade nutrients. Storing fruits and vegetables in the right way helps to retain the nutrients for longer.

All fruits, save for berries (including avocados and tomatoes), should be stored at room temperature and away from direct light

All vegetables, save for the root varieties, should be refrigerated until you use them.

All cut fruits and vegetables should be stored in an airtight container with a dash of lemon juice on them, as Vitamin C, which is an antioxidant, slows down oxidation/decay.

All herbs should be stored chopped up and frozen with water, to preserve their phytonutrients.

Eating raw

The idea behind this is that heating food destroys natural enzymes and nutrients, which is bad as these enzymes help in digestion and also in fighting chronic diseases. So when you cook it, you basically kill it. This diet requires a high level of effort from your end, as the prep work will be extensive. It makes sense to eat most sources of heat-sensitive and water-soluble nutrients raw, as it maximizes the absorption of these nutrients then. For instance, spinach eaten raw provides us with more vitamin C than cooked spinach. Moreover, water-soluble Vitamins C and B are lost when you boil them.

Cooking

However, some foods actually tend to deliver more nutrients when cooked; for example, the lycopene found in tomatoes increases when they are boiled. Similarly, the bioavailability of beta carotene, which is found in carrots, sweet potatoes, spinach, and tomatoes, increases as their plant cell walls are broken down. Cooking denatures the proteins in meat and eggs, making them easier to digest. Iron and other minerals are more available upon cooking as cooking decreases acid oxalates, which otherwise makes these minerals inaccessible, by binding to them.

Moreover, don't overcook your veggies. Using small amounts of water and low heat helps retain their nutrients better. Steaming, sautéing, roasting, blanching, microwaving, and baking are other forms of cooking that you can try.

Chapter 4: Exercise or Diet: What matters more?

Don't be deceived into believing that only dieting will help you shed those extra pounds. Well, it may; however, they won't stay away for long that way. Our body reacts in the same way to starvation and weight loss, that is, by slowing down metabolism, which in turn leads to burning fewer calories. This leads to two things if you continue to consume fewer calories:

A) The weight loss will become slower, or

B) Weight loss will come to a complete halt.

When normal calorie consumption is resumed after this period, you may actually retain more of it as fat and tend to gain more weight than earlier. Moreover, weight loss using this means will tend to increase frailty, especially in older people, because of age-related losses in muscle mass and bone density. The only way to address this is to intensify your physical activity because this will help you counter the metabolic slowdown caused by a reduction in your caloric intake.

If one person increases exercise without cutting back on calories and another one cuts back on calories without exercising, the latter will probably find it easier to shed their weight. This is because it is much easier to reduce 500 calories per day from our diet than it is to burn up 500 calories by exercising. Being active is very important, not just to achieve weight loss; by being active, you burn up more of those calories, and when it is more than you consume, you achieve weight loss.

Exercising regularly helps to increase the amount of energy you burn, as well as boosts the energy expended during resting periods. Resting energy expenditure accounts for 65% to 70% of the calories that you burn each day. Therefore, any increase in this resting energy expenditure is very important in your weight loss journey.

The kinds of physical activities that can help to stimulate your metabolism include riding a bike uphill or walking briskly for a few miles. Even small activities like standing up at your desk instead of being seated constantly can add up to the amount of energy you spend on a daily basis.

Both diet and exercise are equally important. To tell you the truth, diet does have a more prominent effect on weight loss than physical activity. However, the latter has a more lasting and significant effect in preventing this lost weight from returning.

Conclusion

Eat Smart, move more, and live better

Nutrition and lifestyle are key factors in leading a healthy life. Over the course of the book, we have covered different aspects of nutrition and have also taken a look at the different components you will need to include in your diet. You must remember that physical activity and nutrition go hand in hand. Ensure that you get exercise for at least three days a week. I hope you have gathered all the information you were looking for from this book.

Thank you, and remember to share how well these nutrition tips work for you. You can do that by writing a review in your Amazon account under Your Orders > Digital Orders.

Thank you,

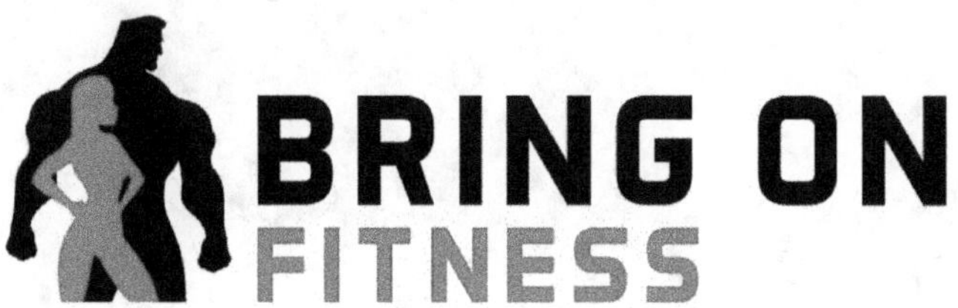